Disclaimer

This book is intended to help people become better informed medical consumers. The information in this book is intended to supplement, not replace, the medical advice of a trained health care professional. No mention or description of uses of drugs listed herein should be construed as an endorsement of those uses or drugs. Only a physician can prescribe drugs and their precise dosages. All matters regarding your health require medical supervision. The authors and publisher disclaim any liability arising directly or indirectly from use of this book.

Notice of rights

Trademarks

Table of Contents

Your feedback is invaluable to us

If you recently bought this book, we would love to hear from you! You can do this by writing a review on amazon (or the online store where you purchased this book) about your last purchase! As part of our continual service improvement process, we love to hear real client experiences and feedback.

How does it work?
To post a review on Amazon, just log in to your account and click on the Create Your Own Review button (under Customer Reviews) of the relevant product page. You can find examples of product reviews in Amazon. If you purchased from another online store, simply follow their procedures.

Why use this book?

Everyone should ask questions when getting a prescription. This is especially important when your doctor or other health care professional prescribes you Mosapride Citrate.

What should you ask?

Your health depends on good communication, but which questions to ask your doctor? Having the right questions is the answer.

Asking questions and providing information to your doctor and other care providers can improve your care. Talking with your doctor builds trust and leads to better satisfaction, quality, safety and results.

Asking questions is key to good communication with your doctor. If you do not ask questions, he or she may assume you already know the answer or that you do not want more information. Do not wait for the doctor to raise a specific question or subject; he or she may not know it is important to you. Be proactive. Ask questions.

Effective health care is a team effort. You are part of this team and play an important role. One of the best ways to communicate with your doctor and health care team is by asking questions. Since time is limited when you have your medical appointments, you will feel less rushed when you prepare your questions before your appointment.

Your doctor wants your questions. Doctors know a lot about a lot of things, but they do not always know everything about you, what you want to know or what is best for you.

Your questions give your doctor and health care professionals important information about you, like your most important health care concerns.

That is why they need you to speak up.

How to use this book?

When you meet with your doctor or other members of your health care team, you will hear a lot of information. It helps to think ahead of time of the things you want to know and to highlight the questions in this book you want to ask and take this book with you to your appointments.

This book contains questions you may want to ask your doctor. You should use the questions that fit your situation, and skip those that do not apply.

This book offers many ways that you can ask questions and get your health care needs met. With this book you will have numerous simple questions that can help you take better care of yourself, feel better, and get the right care at the right time.

Doctors and medical professionals want to know your questions to help them take better care of you and offer advice to get your most pressing questions answered.

Be prepared for your next medical appointment. Take this book with you if you are getting a checkup, want to discuss a problem or health condition, are getting a prescription, or talk about a medical test or surgery and be sure to write down the answers your health care professional provides for you in this book.

Whatever the reason for your appointment, it is important to be prepared.

Take charge of your health. Ask your health care providers questions and learn about the Mosapride Citrate medicine you take.

BEGINNING OF THE
QUESTION CHAPTERS:

CHAPTER #1: WHO:

INTENT: Who benefits from Mosapride
Citrate (Is this right for me.)

1. Please explain, what are the differences between generic and brand Mosapride Citrate medications?

Notes:

2. If the pharmacist offers me a different brand of the same Mosapride Citrate-like medicine - is it ok to take it?

Notes:

3. Who can I contact if I want to meet with a specialist for long-term Mosapride Citrate medication management on an ongoing basis?

Notes:

4. Who gets to see the Mosapride Citrate prescription drug information submitted in my patient medical questionnaire?

Notes:

5. Will my body get to depend upon a certain amount of my Mosapride Citrate prescription drug, an amount that grows higher the longer I am on the drug?

Notes:

6. Do I really need this test?

Notes:

7. Who is accountable for my Mosapride Citrate prescription drug use?

Notes:

8. Would I need Mosapride Citrate prescription drugs that are not covered by insurance?

Notes:

9. Are related potential conditions avoidable, or do they require topical or other prescription medications?

Notes:

10. If I am stranded abroad and run out of my normal Mosapride Citrate prescription medication, am I covered for this?

Notes:

11. Who is eligible to receive Mosapride Citrate prescription drug help?

Notes:

12. Is Mosapride Citrate the right medication?

Notes:

13. When you prescribe Mosapride Citrate prescription medication for my condition, how do you weigh the side effects?

Notes:

14. Do Mosapride Citrate medications work for everybody?

Notes:

15. Can enzymes be taken with other Mosapride Citrate prescription medications?

Notes:

16. Is it probable to uncover how to deal with _____ without taking prescription medication?

Notes:

17. Will Mosapride Citrate meet my expectations?

Notes:

18. How do you help someone who has a Mosapride Citrate prescription drugs addiction?

Notes:

19. May I bring multiple prescription medications to take while I am in custody?

Notes:

20. Can Canadian drug pharmacies mail my Mosapride Citrate prescription drugs and medications to me?

Notes:

21. Who gets Mosapride Citrate, and when?

Notes:

22. Does my condition have to be treated with Mosapride Citrate prescription drugs?

Notes:

23. Is sharing Mosapride Citrate prescription drugs illegal?

Notes:

24. Do I have to pay for my own Mosapride Citrate

prescription drugs?

Notes:

25. Who is qualified to receive Mosapride Citrate prescription drug help?

Notes:

26. When in care who is responsible for the MAR (Medication Administration Records), who can put information on to it and make changes?

Notes:

27. Could any of the Mosapride Citrate medications contribute to impotence?

Notes:

28. Is there an Over-The-Counter Medication that helps or maybe even can replace my Mosapride Citrate Prescription Medication?

Notes:

29. Who makes this Mosapride Citrate medication?

Notes:

30. Do you know all of the risks Mosapride Citrate prescription drugs might pose?

Notes:

31. Who is most susceptible to Mosapride Citrate prescription drug abuse?

Notes:

32. Are there simpler - safer options?

Notes:

33. Who should NOT take Mosapride Citrate medication?

Notes:

34. Who can get Medicare Mosapride Citrate prescription drug coverage?

Notes:

35. Can we really know what is in Mosapride Citrate prescription drugs?

Notes:

36. Is there anything I can do on my own to improve my condition?

Notes:

37. Will Mosapride Citrate prescription medications cause weight loss?

Notes:

38. Is it likely to get worse, or is it likely to get better?

Notes:

39. Will any tests be necessary while I am taking Mosapride Citrate medication?

Notes:

40. Are there any other precautions or warnings for this Mosapride Citrate medication?

Notes:

41. Who can assist with Mosapride Citrate medication reminders?

Notes:

42. Can alternative medicine counter Mosapride Citrate prescription medication and over-the-counters with their limited effectiveness and potential side effects?

Notes:

43. How to get my Mosapride Citrate medication increased?

Notes:

44. How do you prevent re-admission in case I forget to take my Mosapride Citrate prescription medications. How do you help those who have

problems following suggestions regarding eating habits, smoking, drinking, and taking drugs..?

Notes:

45. Does my plan cover my Mosapride Citrate prescription drugs?

Notes:

46. Can all doctors prescribe Mosapride Citrate Prescription Medication?

Notes:

47. What is the Prescription Drug Monitoring Database and who is using it?

Notes:

48. Could natural products be just as effective as Mosapride Citrate prescription medications?

Notes:

49. Are there any drug interactions if Mosapride

Citrate is taken in combination with other medications?

Notes:

50. Do you know of any medications available out there that would help me be more comfortable?

Notes:

51. Who typically uses Mosapride Citrate prescription drugs, and where do they get them?

Notes:

52. Do I HAVE to be on Mosapride Citrate medication?

Notes:

53. How can I get Mosapride Citrate prescription drug coverage?

Notes:

54. What can I expect about the absorption of active ingredients in my Mosapride Citrate prescription

medications?

Notes:

55. What if I am out of the country and lose my Mosapride Citrate prescription medications?

Notes:

56. Can a Mosapride Citrate prescription drug card preserve me cash?

Notes:

57. Who is validating my Mosapride Citrate prescription drugs to make sure I am taking the correct pills?

Notes:

58. How can you help me when I suffer from chronic pain, but am leery about taking prescription medication to help it?

Notes:

59. What is your opinion on Mosapride Citrate prescription medications , side effects and IBS?

Notes:

60. What would happen if I were suddenly unable to get access to my Mosapride Citrate prescription drugs?

Notes:

61. Is Mosapride Citrate a medication?

Notes:

62. Is this worth getting Mosapride Citrate medication for?

Notes:

63. If I want to talk to a specialist in Mosapride Citrate prescription drugs, where do I go?

Notes:

64. Who can join a Medicare Mosapride Citrate

prescription drug plan?

Notes:

65. If I am unable to comply with the treatment regimen, who else can administer Mosapride Citrate medication?

Notes:

66. Who is at risk for Mosapride Citrate prescription drug addiction?

Notes:

67. Can you help me save money on my Mosapride Citrate prescription medication?

Notes:

68. Can you suggest alternatives to Mosapride Citrate prescription medication?

Notes:

69. Can using too much or too little Mosapride Citrate

prescription drugs harm my health?

Notes:

70. Do individual policies pay for prescription Mosapride Citrate medications?

Notes:

71. What is the difference between brand name medication and their generic counter parts?

Notes:

72. Um - can you explain that again?

Notes:

73. What is the safest prescription drug disposal method?

Notes:

74. Is Mosapride Citrate medication a substitute for therapy?

Notes:

75. Can my baby get harmed by my Mosapride Citrate prescription drug use?

Notes:

76. What treatments, therapies and medications are recommended or available for my condition?

Notes:

77. Do we have to do this now - or can we revisit it later?

Notes:

78. Has there been any follow up of those who have stopped taking Mosapride Citrate medication?

Notes:

79. Is it safe and legal to buy Mosapride Citrate prescription drugs and other medications abroad?

Notes:

80. What if my religion condones the use of Mosapride Citrate medications?

Notes:

81. Should I expect a dependance on a medication which provides relief?

Notes:

82. Do I need a change in my Mosapride Citrate medication?

Notes:

83. How can a wholesome mud-bath help my condition, and what is the effect on my Mosapride Citrate prescription drugs?

Notes:

84. What if my current Mosapride Citrate prescription drugs are not on the formulary or are limited on the formulary?

Notes:

85. Is Mosapride Citrate addictive?

Notes:

86. Is there a better way to easily adhere to Mosapride Citrate prescription medication regimens?

Notes:

87. Can I ever be free of having to use prescription drugs?

Notes:

88. What are generic alternatives for my Mosapride Citrate prescription drugs?

Notes:

89. Will Mosapride Citrate interact with my current medications?

Notes:

90. Is there an effective herbal alternative or supplement to Mosapride Citrate medication?

Notes:

91. So who approves these Mosapride Citrate medications?

Notes:

92. What do each of these Mosapride Citrate prescription medications have in common?

Notes:

93. Will you try and reach the primary reason for my problem before prescribing Mosapride Citrate medications to solve my particular signs and symptoms?

Notes:

CHAPTER #2: WHAT:

INTENT: What do I need to know about
Mosapride Citrate (What will it do for
me and what can I expect.)

1. What exactly leads one to get dependent on
Mosapride Citrate prescription drugs?

Notes:

2. What about taking a new Mosapride Citrate
medication?

Notes:

3. What Mosapride Citrate's class medication can I take
best?

Notes:

4. What are other treatment options?

Notes:

5. What is the brand name for the drug Mosapride Citrate?

Notes:

6. What other sources are available, who can I talk to about this?

Notes:

7. What will a positive result mean?

Notes:

8. What could be a natural alternative to more over-the-counter and Mosapride Citrate prescription drugs?

Notes:

9. What does my Mosapride Citrate medication look like?

Notes:

10. What Mosapride Citrate prescription drugs have serious side effects?

Notes:

11. What is my Mosapride Citrate prescription drug benefit?

Notes:

12. Can you help me understand how much of my Mosapride Citrate prescription drugs, equipment and services will be covered by my insurance and what I will have to pay?

Notes:

13. What if the Mosapride Citrate medications produce unwelcome or harmful effects?

Notes:

14. What are the important warnings for females taking Mosapride Citrate?

Notes:

15. What types of Mosapride Citrate medications are available?

Notes:

16. What is the test for?

Notes:

17. What if I am unhappy with the results of Mosapride Citrate medication?

Notes:

18. What about my current medications or allergies and the effect on it of Mosapride Citrate?

Notes:

19. What about my regular medications, any

interference with Mosapride Citrate?

Notes:

20. What medications should I ask for?

Notes:

21. What about Mosapride Citrate prescription drug coverage?

Notes:

22. What are the causes of Mosapride Citrate prescription drug abuse?

Notes:

23. What's the best mix for me of home remedies, over the counter (OTC) drugs and ointments and Mosapride Citrate prescription drugs?

Notes:

24. What's next?

Notes:

25. What's the difference between all of the Mosapride Citrate's class medications?

Notes:

26. What sort of Mosapride Citrate prescription drug benefit is included?

Notes:

27. What are the adverse health effects from Mosapride Citrate prescription drugs?

Notes:

28. What is the safest way to dispose of unwanted medications?

Notes:

29. What is the nature of the Mosapride Citrate medications prescribed?

Notes:

30. What can parents and other adults do to help prevent prescription drug abuse among youth?

Notes:

31. What if my prescription Mosapride Citrate medication is lost or stolen?

Notes:

32. What medications can Mosapride Citrate interact with?

Notes:

33. What are my options in relation to Mosapride Citrate medication, surgical procedures or remedy?

Notes:

34. What are the side effects?

Notes:

35. Apart from Mosapride Citrate medication, what are other components of your management plan?

Notes:

36. What Mosapride Citrate medications are used?

Notes:

37. What's your go-to question for your own doctor?

Notes:

38. What are the Mosapride Citrate medication side-effects?

Notes:

39. What should I do if I have other prescription drug coverage and want to join Medicare First?

Notes:

40. What side effects can Mosapride Citrate

medication cause?

Notes:

41. What is the branded prescription drug fee?

Notes:

42. What medications on the market, OTC or Mosapride Citrate prescription, can become harmful over time and would be dangerous if used well past the expiration date?

Notes:

43. What are the different treatment options?

Notes:

44. What are my Mosapride Citrate medication options?

Notes:

45. What are the side effects of the Mosapride Citrate medication?

Notes:

46. What is the name of my Mosapride Citrate medication?

Notes:

47. What sources can I trust?

Notes:

48. What's to lose by trying another Mosapride Citrate class medication?

Notes:

49. What is the safest way to dispose of unused prescription Mosapride Citrate medication?

Notes:

50. What if I'm already on medication and have side-effects from the Mosapride Citrate?

Notes:

51. What is Mosapride Citrate prescription drug detox?

Notes:

52. What if I have tried various home remedies, over-the-counter medications or even Mosapride Citrate prescription medications with no help?

Notes:

53. What should I do if I experience side effects from the Mosapride Citrate?

Notes:

54. What outcome should I expect?

Notes:

55. What will a negative result mean?

Notes:

56. What other drugs could interact with Mosapride Citrate medication?

Notes:

57. What Mosapride Citrate medication should I take?

Notes:

58. What does a Mosapride Citrate medication error involve?

Notes:

59. Is treatment required, if so - what is it?

Notes:

60. What are the important warnings for males taking Mosapride Citrate?

Notes:

61. What is a 25/50 percent Mosapride Citrate prescription drug plan?

Notes:

62. What are your experiences with Mosapride Citrate prescription drugs?

Notes:

63. What kind of experience with these issues do you have?

Notes:

64. What if I have been taking Mosapride Citrate medication with little to no relief?

Notes:

65. What happens if I don't do anything?

Notes:

66. What if Mosapride Citrate medication has changed since the application form was sent in?

Notes:

67. Will I need medication and what will it be, Mosapride Citrate and/or anything else?

Notes:

68. What if I take Mosapride Citrate prescription drugs and get little or no relief?

Notes:

69. How do scientists determine whether the chemical compounds in Mosapride Citrate prescription medications do what they're claimed to do?

Notes:

70. What happens if I stop using Mosapride Citrate cold-turkey?

Notes:

71. At what point would you recommend Mosapride Citrate prescription drugs, alternative therapies, or surgery?

Notes:

72. What about side effects of Mosapride Citrate?

Notes:

73. What are your thoughts on hypnotherapy and Mosapride Citrate?

Notes:

74. What if Mosapride Citrate medication makes me gain weight?

Notes:

75. What is the way to get my life back on track, without the unwanted side effects of Mosapride Citrate prescription drugs?

Notes:

76. What if I am taking vitamins or over-the-counter drugs that could affect my Mosapride Citrate prescription drugs?

Notes:

77. What if I am currently taking some other prescription medications?

Notes:

78. What can I do to help win the war on prescription drug abuse?

Notes:

79. What will this test tell us?

Notes:

80. What really works as well as these Mosapride Citrate medications, are there alternatives?

Notes:

81. Is Mosapride Citrate safe when breastfeeding, what are the effects on nursing?

Notes:

82. What causes my condition?

Notes:

83. What is are food or drinks you recommend not to be taken with Mosapride Citrate prescription medications?

Notes:

84. What sexual response side effects can I expect from these Mosapride Citrate medications?

Notes:

85. What are my options if I have difficulty paying for Mosapride Citrate prescription drugs?

Notes:

86. What are my risks of accidentally taking an overdose of Mosapride Citrate prescription drugs?

Notes:

87. What are the signs and symptoms related to Mosapride Citrate addiction?

Notes:

88. What kind of Mosapride Citrate medications do the varying plans offer and how much can I save?

Notes:

89. What is the best approach if I forget to take this Mosapride Citrate medication?

Notes:

90. What would you do if you were me?

Notes:

91. What happens with my prescriptions for Mosapride Citrate medications while I am travelling overseas, how to get and fulfil those?

Notes:

92. What prescription medications or off the shelf medicinal products would cause ringing in the ears?

Notes:

93. What else could I be doing to stay healthy and prevent disease?

Notes:

94. What kind of resources do I have available to me?

Notes:

95. What are some of the best non prescription medications I can give a try?

Notes:

96. I want to read more about my condition. What online sources should I trust?

Notes:

97. What is Mosapride Citrate medication for?

Notes:

98. What is a generic Mosapride Citrate medication?

Notes:

99. What lifestyle changes can change my condition?

Notes:

100. What do I need to know about making the most of this Mosapride Citrate prescription?

Notes:

101. What will be the net effect of Mosapride Citrate medications for me?

Notes:

102. What can I do to prevent my condition from recurring or worsening?

Notes:

103. What about alcohol and its effect on Mosapride Citrate prescription drugs?

Notes:

104. What medications are available to treat my condition?

Notes:

105. What are good reasons to not take my Mosapride Citrate prescription medication?

Notes:

106. What replacement medications can you suggest for Mosapride Citrate?

Notes:

107. How do I book in to have the test and what is the usual waiting period?

Notes:

108. What else can I do to treat my condition?

Notes:

109. What will happen to me without Mosapride Citrate prescription drugs, diet, exercise, or nutritional supplements?

Notes:

110. Besides Mosapride Citrate medication, what else to do?

Notes:

111. What is the name of my condition, are there any other names it's known by?

Notes:

112. What is a generic Mosapride Citrate medication or drug, what does that term mean and what can it do for me?

Notes:

113. What about Mosapride Citrate's interactions with my medications?

Notes:

114. What is my outcome?

Notes:

115. What can I do to remember to take my Mosapride Citrate medication?

Notes:

116. What non-Mosapride Citrate medications or vitamins should I take to speed up my healing?

Notes:

117. What is the proper course of treatment for me?

Notes:

118. For what reasons would I have to be off Mosapride Citrate medication and for how long?

Notes:

119. What are the dosages of the Mosapride Citrate medication?

Notes:

120. What types of vitamins and supplements should I be taking?

Notes:

121. What medications have you yourself used in the past to make yourself better?

Notes:

122. What will happen if I don't have the treatment?

Notes:

123. What if I'm taking other medication?

Notes:

124. What happens if I have to cut my Mosapride Citrate pills in half to make them last longer or skip a day of medication because I can't afford to buy it as often as it's prescribed?

Notes:

125. What to eat, or what to use as a medication together with Mosapride Citrate?

Notes:

126. What is the easiest way to obtain the latest information about Mosapride Citrate prescription drugs?

Notes:

127. What is a prescription drug error and how often and why do these errors occur??

Notes:

128. What do you recommend to do with Mosapride Citrate medication adherence being difficult for me since my busy life pulls me in multiple directions - can you help me understand the ramifications of non-adherence?

Notes:

129. In what way can mindfulness or meditation be useful?

Notes:

130. What is the evidence for this treatment?

Notes:

131. What are the Mosapride Citrate medications I can take?

Notes:

132. What are the benefits of having the test?

Notes:

133. What other Mosapride Citrate-like medications are in this class?

Notes:

134. What questions haven't I asked that I should have?

Notes:

135. What should I expect after a procedure in terms of soreness, what to watch for, Mosapride Citrate medication, bathing, and level of activity?

Notes:

136. What should you, as my doctor, know before prescribing Mosapride Citrate medication?

Notes:

137. What will my Mosapride Citrate medication do for me?

Notes:

138. What kind of expectations should I have?

Notes:

139. What should I do if I miss my regular dose of Mosapride Citrate?

Notes:

140. Is it possible that my employer may look at what Mosapride Citrate prescription medications I'm taking?

Notes:

141. What is the prescription drug of choice for breakthrough pain meds?

Notes:

142. Do I need to change what I eat or stop any Mosapride Citrate medications before doing a test?

Notes:

143. How will you know what medications I am on?

Notes:

144. What can I expect from Mosapride Citrate medication?

Notes:

145. In what situation would I need to go for counseling if I'm receiving medication treatment?

Notes:

146. What does this sign on my Mosapride Citrate prescription drug imply?

Notes:

147. What prescription drugs are you yourself taking?

Notes:

148. What is the effect of Mosapride Citrate on infertility?

Notes:

149. How will I benefit from working out in relation to my use of Mosapride Citrate prescription medication, and what type of exercise would you recommend?

Notes:

150. What Mosapride Citrate-like medications are safe to take during pregnancy?

Notes:

151. What other prescription drugs should I avoid while taking my Mosapride Citrate medicines?

Notes:

152. What would happen if I don't take the Mosapride Citrate, would my health get worse?

Notes:

153. What kind of medication will I have to take, Mosapride Citrate or anything else?

Notes:

154. What's the probability that my Mosapride Citrate medication is causing my symptoms?

Notes:

155. What is the effect of Mosapride Citrate on drowsiness?

Notes:

156. What if I have an allergic reaction to Mosapride Citrate?

Notes:

157. What should I know about Mosapride Citrate medication?

Notes:

CHAPTER #3: WHERE:

INTENT: Where to next (Where can I find more information. Do i need a second opionion. What happens with tests.)

1. Is there a possibility of reaction to Mosapride Citrate medications?

Notes:

2. Where are others buying their Mosapride Citrate prescription medications?

Notes:

3. Where I can get a Mosapride Citrate prescription drug?

Notes:

4. Can Mosapride Citrate medication cause hair loss?

Notes:

5. Is the answer in natural supplements, in Mosapride Citrate prescription medications or some combination of both?

Notes:

6. Do you offer treatment programs for those suffering from Mosapride Citrate prescription drug addiction?

Notes:

7. Can people be guilty of DUI if they are driving under the influence of Mosapride Citrate prescription medications?

Notes:

8. What does using a prescription drug Off-label mean?

Notes:

9. Could you write it down?

Notes:

10. What is a 3-Tier or 4-Tier prescription drug plan?

Notes:

11. Is this normal or should I see a shrink for Mosapride Citrate medication?

Notes:

12. Can I expect any side effects from my Mosapride Citrate medication?

Notes:

13. Where do I go if I've run out of money and desperately need Mosapride Citrate medication or a medical procedure?

Notes:

14. Will I require any Mosapride Citrate prescription drugs?

Notes:

15. Should I take my Mosapride Citrate medications at a regular time each day?

Notes:

16. I'm taking prescription medication abroad, will this be covered if it is lost or I run out?

Notes:

17. Can I take Mosapride Citrate with my other medications?

Notes:

18. Are Mosapride Citrate prescription drugs covered?

Notes:

19. Do vitamins interact with Mosapride Citrate

medications?

Notes:

20. Are you aware of my personal medical history including current medications, allergies, and other considerations or limitations?

Notes:

21. Can I take Mosapride Citrate medication?

Notes:

22. Are non-prescription drugs less effective than Mosapride Citrate?

Notes:

23. Should I stop taking that Mosapride Citrate medication?

Notes:

24. Does it matter at what time I use my Mosapride Citrate medication?

Notes:

25. Is it true that an online pharmacy can save me money on Mosapride Citrate prescription drugs?

Notes:

26. Where would I store my Mosapride Citrate medications?

Notes:

27. Can you slow down and keep it simple?

Notes:

28. Is there anything I can do to improve it myself?

Notes:

29. Which Mosapride Citrate's class related medication is the safest for me?

Notes:

30. Are any medications I am taking likely to cause breast problems?

Notes:

31. What happens if I am willing to try new medications if the current Mosapride Citrate ones are not working?

Notes:

32. Can I share Mosapride Citrate prescription drugs?

Notes:

33. Should I have a current emergency contact form and a list of health conditions and medications readily available?

Notes:

34. Where can I buy Mosapride Citrate prescription drugs cheaper?

Notes:

35. Will taking Mosapride Citrate make me irritable?

Notes:

36. Will Mosapride Citrate prescriptions drugs affect urine drug screen?

Notes:

37. Which Mosapride Citrate prescription drugs can be addictive?

Notes:

38. Do you think that I may have or get a problem with Mosapride Citrate medications?

Notes:

39. Will I be able to carry enough prescription medications to avoid any health emergencies?

Notes:

40. What kinds of medications will I need to take and what if they don't work?

Notes:

41. Are there any side effects of taking Mosapride Citrate?

41. Are there any side effects of taking Mosapride Citrate?

Notes:

42. Do I need to see any other health professionals - such as specialists - physiotherapists - dieticians or dentists?

Notes:

43. Are you considering a trial of Mosapride Citrate medications and/or anything else?

Notes:

44. Is there anything else I should be asking?

Notes:

45. Should I buy generic Mosapride Citrate

prescription medications?

Notes:

46. Do I really need to take this Mosapride Citrate medication?

Notes:

47. Where should I get my Mosapride Citrate prescription drugs?

Notes:

48. Will you try and keep my Mosapride Citrate medications at a level where I can function?

Notes:

49. Do pill boxes help prevent Mosapride Citrate medication errors?

Notes:

50. Because Medicare prescription drug coverage is so new to me, where can I get aid deciding on a

program?

Notes:

51. Should I be concerned about all the Mosapride Citrate medication I need to take to stay on top of my health problems?

Notes:

52. Does my plan have a Mosapride Citrate prescription drug formulary?

Notes:

53. Is it okay to take my Mosapride Citrate prescription drugs and multivitamin during a fast?

Notes:

54. Should I lock up my Mosapride Citrate prescription drugs?

Notes:

55. Is my weight okay?

Notes:

56. Is it possible to start with a solution which is natural and effective and less expensive than Mosapride Citrate prescription medication?

Notes:

57. Can the nurse see me?

Notes:

58. How do I avoid getting in a place where I need so many prescription drugs to function?

Notes:

59. Will Mosapride Citrate have an effect on nausea?

Notes:

60. Will Mosapride Citrate cause me to test positive for various substances in a urine drug test?

Notes:

61. Are my Mosapride Citrate prescription drugs FDA-approved?

Notes:

62. Where can I get my Mosapride Citrate prescription medications filled?

Notes:

63. Would increasing the dose of Mosapride Citrate have a positive effect or would I be better off asking you to try some new medications?

Notes:

64. Where can US citizens buy their prescription drugs online from legally, in confidence, and under which conditions?

Notes:

65. Do I need to take Mosapride Citrate medications?

Notes:

66. Can Mosapride Citrate be mixed with other medications, dietary supplements, or alcohol?

Notes:

67. If there is an all new Mosapride Citrate medication that comes up how can it have been adequately tested in terms of it's long term negative effects?

Notes:

68. Are there less intrusive, harmless and effective solutions instead of Mosapride Citrate prescription drugs?

Notes:

69. Can you inform me about nutrition, exercise, Mosapride Citrate medications and complications?

Notes:

70. Can I take over-the-counter drugs or are prescription drugs more effective?

Notes:

71. Does Mosapride Citrate medication and therapy work together?

Notes:

72. Should I take Mosapride Citrate medication or explore alternative natural treatments?

Notes:

73. How can I legally purchase Mosapride Citrate prescription medications from Canada?

Notes:

74. Do I have to be on more medications because of the side effects of Mosapride Citrate?

Notes:

75. If I use prescription drugs, can I be arrested for DUI?

Notes:

76. Do I need to prepare for the test (for example - by fasting beforehand)?

Notes:

77. Where can I get more info about that?

Notes:

78. Should I rely on Mosapride Citrate, natural cures or over the counter medication?

Notes:

79. If remedies help, what is the nature of Mosapride Citrate medications and where could one go to explore them?

Notes:

80. Does my policy cover Mosapride Citrate prescription drugs?

Notes:

81. Where would you send your partner or children?

Notes:

82. Who monitors the safety and effectiveness of Mosapride Citrate prescription drugs?

Notes:

83. Is it normal to feel this way?

Notes:

84. Are the supplements I take worthwhile?

Notes:

85. Where can I find info about taking more than one prescription medications together with Mosapride Citrate?

Notes:

86. Should I get a second opinion?

Notes:

87. What are the best ways that do not require prescription medications to fall asleep faster?

Notes:

88. Do I need any Mosapride Citrate medications?

Notes:

89. What are the Mosapride Citrate prescription drug prices?

Notes:

90. Do I need medication or surgery?

Notes:

91. Are there any alternative tests?

Notes:

92. Are Mosapride Citrate medications toxic?

Notes:

93. Which one of Mosapride Citrate medications is better for me than the others?

Notes:

CHAPTER #4: WHEN:

INTENT: When should I take or stop taking Mosapride Citrate and how (When should I take it, stop taking it and how.)

1. Is there any form of exercise or medication you can recommend to enhance the effects of Mosapride Citrate?

Notes:

2. Are there any known Mosapride Citrate prescription medication and chia seeds side effects when they are combined?

Notes:

3. If I could possibly reduce the number of prescription drugs besides Mosapride Citrate I have

to take for various conditions and feel a lot better by taking a single substance, would you look into it?

Notes:

4. Should I take Mosapride Citrate with other medications?

Notes:

5. Do enzymes interfere with Mosapride Citrate prescription drugs?

Notes:

6. Is switching from one biologic medication to another effective?

Notes:

7. How does herb _____ compare to, or has an effect on, Mosapride Citrate prescription drugs?

Notes:

8. When should I stop taking Mosapride Citrate

medication?

Notes:

9. What are some great ways to help remind me when to take Mosapride Citrate medications?

Notes:

10. Should I bring my Mosapride Citrate medications with me everywhere I go?

Notes:

11. Is it either / or when it comes to natural medicines and Mosapride Citrate prescription drugs?

Notes:

12. Will I have to take my medications forever?

Notes:

13. Can you help me with finding the money to purchase doctor visits and also Mosapride Citrate prescriptions medication?

Notes:

14. Can I take Mosapride Citrate with other medications?

Notes:

15. What should I consider when buying coverage that provides prescription drug benefits?

Notes:

16. When will I know that I am taking excessive pain medication?

Notes:

17. When I have been on the same amount of Mosapride Citrate medication for years – when should that be re-evaluated?

Notes:

18. How do I deal with any Mosapride Citrate prescription medication when a side effect may be

stated as 'may cause nausea or vomiting'?

Notes:

19. Will I get possible side neuritis of Mosapride Citrate medications?

Notes:

20. What is the difference between a natural herbal supplement and a prescription drug?

Notes:

21. Are there any contraindications with Mosapride Citrate to other medications?

Notes:

22. How/when do I get test results?

Notes:

23. Is Mosapride Citrate medication the only answer for me?

Notes:

24. Is there a generic version of the Mosapride Citrate medication?

Notes:

25. Will I feel doped from Mosapride Citrate?

Notes:

26. Is this necessary now?

Notes:

27. Should I stop my Mosapride Citrate medications before any procedure?

Notes:

28. So, are Mosapride Citrate prescription drugs safe?

Notes:

29. Do Mosapride Citrate prescription drugs create new mental problems?

Notes:

30. What if I refuse the prescribed Mosapride Citrate medication?

Notes:

31. When might herbal and nutritional therapies be a good alternative to over-the-counter and Mosapride Citrate prescription medications for people with my condition?

Notes:

32. Mosapride Citrate is most definitely a prescription drug?

Notes:

33. Are side effects from Mosapride Citrate medications the same in males and females?

Notes:

34. What prescription drugs do I need covered?

Notes:

35. What medications do I need to stop and when?

Notes:

36. Can the Mosapride Citrate medication cause substance abuse?

Notes:

37. Should I stop taking my Mosapride Citrate medication(s) before a evaluation or a surgery?

Notes:

38. Will my Mosapride Citrate prescription drugs build up toxins in my body?

Notes:

39. When could Mosapride Citrate medication not be working anymore?

Notes:

40. If you have a Mosapride Citrate prescription drug in your pocket, outside of the container when arrested is that considered DUI?

Notes:

41. What medications are safe for me to take during my pregnancy?

Notes:

42. What does 50 deductible for brand name prescription drugs mean?

Notes:

43. When did you graduate from medical school?

Notes:

44. Will any supplements interact with my Mosapride Citrate prescription drugs?

Notes:

45. Do you have my vital records and medications up to date?

Notes:

46. How do Mosapride Citrate prescription drugs work?

Notes:

47. Will I be able to take my prescription medications after surgery?

Notes:

48. When is it appropriate and safe to prescribe Mosapride Citrate medication for my condition?

Notes:

49. If I take Mosapride Citrate prescription drugs long term, do I run the risk of becoming addicted?

Notes:

50. How long am I expected to take this Mosapride Citrate medication?

Notes:

51. What if I start depending on antidepressants, alcohol, or other medications to calm me down or help me sleep?

Notes:

52. When does Mosapride Citrate medication begin working?

Notes:

53. Will I be on Mosapride Citrate medication forever?

Notes:

54. What is the effect of my Mosapride Citrate use if I smoke?

Notes:

55. May my employer ask me which Mosapride Citrate prescription medications I am taking?

Notes:

56. When should I stop using Mosapride Citrate medication because of....?

Notes:

57. Do you earn bonuses based on performance?

Notes:

58. How do I use my insurance to get discounts on my Mosapride Citrate prescription medication?

Notes:

59. Does Mosapride Citrate medication work?

Notes:

60. How and when should I take my Mosapride Citrate

medication?

Notes:

61. Will Mosapride Citrate prescription medications cause gum problems?

Notes:

62. Can Reiki be used when taking Mosapride Citrate medications?

Notes:

63. Are there medications available that really fix the underlying cause of my condition?

Notes:

64. Can this test diagnose a problem or will I need further testing?

Notes:

65. Could Mosapride Citrate prescription medications cause a false positive on a test?

Notes:

66. Do you know of any natural medication to help?

Notes:

67. Are the brands of Mosapride Citrate prescription drugs I take covered?

Notes:

68. Is there a certain Mosapride Citrate or other medication that can improve my symptoms?

Notes:

69. When should I take this Mosapride Citrate medicine?

Notes:

70. Can assisted living patients receive 90-day supplies of medications?

Notes:

71. Can I schedule my surgery for the morning?

Notes:

72. When does this Mosapride Citrate medication expire?

Notes:

73. Is _____ a side effect of Mosapride Citrate medication and is it permanent?

Notes:

74. When should I be on Mosapride Citrate medication?

Notes:

75. What should you do if I've messed up with my Mosapride Citrate medication?

Notes:

76. Where else can I go for Mosapride Citrate prescription medication, what are my options?

Notes:

77. Is there an effective way to prevent and treat without Mosapride Citrate prescription drugs?

Notes:

78. Precisely what are some good reasons Mosapride Citrate prescription drugs can be recommended?

Notes:

79. Should I really use this Mosapride Citrate medication?

Notes:

80. Can I take Mosapride Citrate with my current medications?

Notes:

81. Do you have research you can share on Mosapride Citrate prescription drug prices?

Notes:

82. Are there any side effects from taking nutritional supplements and Mosapride Citrate prescription medications at the same time?

Notes:

83. Is there anything I should do to help prevent my health issue?

Notes:

84. When and how will I get the results?

Notes:

85. How does my child at an out-of-state school obtain prescription drugs?

Notes:

86. Can you take expired Mosapride Citrate medications or not?

Notes:

87. What herbs, supplements, foods, drinks or activities should I avoid while taking Mosapride Citrate medication?

Notes:

88. When can seniors join a Mosapride Citrate prescription drug plan?

Notes:

89. Is self-administration of Mosapride Citrate medication allowed?

Notes:

90. Will Mosapride Citrate medication be the proper strength?

Notes:

91. Will I need any Mosapride Citrate medication after surgery?

Notes:

92. What does one do when the only real help, the only Mosapride Citrate medication available, no longer works?

Notes:

93. Common side effects of Mosapride Citrate include?

Notes:

CHAPTER #5: WHY:

INTENT: Why do I need Mosapride Citrate (Are there Alternatives. Why do I need it. Which symptoms does it medicate.)

1. Is it possible to lower my blood pressure without taking prescription drugs?

Notes:

2. Will my gender or ethnic group be denied Mosapride Citrate medications that work better for other groups but not for my ethnic or gender group?

Notes:

3. Why would I, while regularly taking prescription medications, have to approach grapefruit consumption with caution?

Notes:

4. Should I be worried about this lump/spot/_____?

Notes:

5. Does my health insurance plan provide prescription drug benefits?

Notes:

6. Are any medications I am taking dangerous for my stage of this disease?

Notes:

7. Which Mosapride Citrate medications are addictive?

Notes:

8. Should I eat while taking specialized Mosapride Citrate prescription drugs?

Notes:

9. Can I take ayurvedic products with Mosapride Citrate prescription medications?

Notes:

10. Can nutritional yeasts, especially brewers yeast, interact with Mosapride Citrate medications?

Notes:

11. What are the differences between generic and brand medications?

Notes:

12. Why would I need Mosapride Citrate prescription medication reminders?

Notes:

13. Why does my family's medical history matter, and what should I do about it?

Notes:

14. Can Mosapride Citrate prescription drugs cause problems during pregnancy?

Notes:

15. Where does my Mosapride Citrate prescription medication come from?

Notes:

16. Are all Mosapride Citrate prescription drugs covered under health care plans?

Notes:

17. How do I get my Mosapride Citrate medication without prescription drug coverage?

Notes:

18. Will St. John's Wort interfere with Mosapride Citrate prescription medications?

Notes:

19. Is it all right for me to take allergy medication?

Notes:

20. Does the Mosapride Citrate medicine need to be stored in the fridge?

Notes:

21. Has anyone ever used this Mosapride Citrate medication?

Notes:

22. Will any of the current Mosapride Citrate medications I am taking increase my risk for _____?

Notes:

23. Do Mosapride Citrate medications accelerate aging?

Notes:

24. Why are we doing these tests?

Notes:

25. Can I take _____ with Mosapride Citrate prescription drugs?

Notes:

26. Do Mosapride Citrate medications deliver on their promise?

Notes:

27. Where can I make cost savings?

Notes:

28. Are there health insurers who reimburse for Mosapride Citrate prescription drugs based on how well they work?

Notes:

29. Why have my bowel habits/appetite/mood/sex drive/etc changed?

Notes:

30. Are there other remedies, is there any relief other than Mosapride Citrate Medication?

Notes:

31. Why is this Mosapride Citrate medication prescribed?

Notes:

32. Which method of Mosapride Citrate prescription medication detox is best?

Notes:

33. What if I am affected by anxiety and don't like the thought of taking prescription medications?

Notes:

34. Are there any co-pays for medical treatments, hospitalization or Mosapride Citrate prescription drugs?

Notes:

35. If I have been taking the same prescription drugs for a long time, when is it time to evaluate?

Notes:

36. Do I need this particular Mosapride Citrate medication?

Notes:

37. Are generics available for all Mosapride Citrate prescription drugs?

Notes:

38. Why is it important to take my Mosapride Citrate prescription medication exactly as prescribed?

Notes:

39. Which Mosapride Citrate-related prescription drugs are most dangerous?

Notes:

40. Why do I need Mosapride Citrate medicine?

Notes:

41. Why does a prescription drug require authorization by a qualified professional and others do not?

Notes:

42. Is there a non-prescription Mosapride Citrate medication you might recommend?

Notes:

43. Why are you giving me a blood test - and what will the results tell us?

Notes:

44. Will Mosapride Citrate interfere with other prescription medications?

Notes:

45. Are there any other medicines that can help me but without any side effects?

Notes:

46. Could a lot of the symptoms and brain fog I get be from the Mosapride Citrate medications themselves?

Notes:

47. Can my condition come back?

Notes:

48. Why is Mosapride Citrate medication prescribed?

Notes:

49. Do you have Mosapride Citrate prescription drugs I can take throughout the day?

Notes:

50. How do you handle potential prescription drug addiction and flow-on depression?

Notes:

51. Is it safe getting pregnant while on Mosapride Citrate medications?

Notes:

52. When is it time to think about why I'm on these Mosapride Citrate drugs?

Notes:

53. Why are you doing this test?

Notes:

54. What f I have any allergies to food, medications or things in the environment?

Notes:

55. Do younger people need less of the Mosapride Citrate medication than older people?

Notes:

56. Why can't I buy some prescription drugs online?

Notes:

57. Why and when use acupuncture for treating pain instead of, or combined with, taking pain medication?

Notes:

58. Why is Mosapride Citrate a prescription drug?

Notes:

59. How do I safely discard Mosapride Citrate prescription drugs without having to worry?

Notes:

60. Where can I obtain a list of Mosapride Citrate prescription drugs that require prior approval?

Notes:

61. I feel like I need more medication, will you as my doctor be able to support me with my requests?

Notes:

62. Are Mosapride Citrate prescription medications included in my monthly insurance fee?

Notes:

63. Should I bring a list of medications and allergies?

Notes:

64. Are Mosapride Citrate medications effective?

Notes:

65. Are extended-release (ER) opioid medications optimum pain medications?

Notes:

66. Can I safely use natural remedies and Mosapride Citrate prescription drugs together?

Notes:

67. Should I be on Mosapride Citrate medication?

Notes:

68. If I get concerned with the high cost of medical care and Mosapride Citrate prescriptions drugs, will you help me explore my options for a more natural approach like seeking help from acupuncturists, naturopaths, chiropractors?

Notes:

69. How to take Mosapride Citrate medication?

Notes:

70. Is this something I should worry about or is it just a side effect of Mosapride Citrate?

Notes:

71. Why do I need to manage Mosapride Citrate medications?

Notes:

72. What if I am currently without prescription drug coverage?

Notes:

73. Did you wash your hands?

Notes:

74. Are there safe Mosapride Citrate-class prescription drugs available?

Notes:

75. If I am taking Mosapride Citrate prescription medications can I take natural remedies?

Notes:

76. Is Mosapride Citrate a medicine with real

evidence?

Notes:

77. Have you heard any stories about buying Mosapride Citrate prescription drugs over the internet?

Notes:

78. If I take a Mosapride Citrate medication, will it require more medication to counter the side effects?

Notes:

79. Are there any side effects associated with this Mosapride Citrate medication that I should know about?

Notes:

80. Where are Mosapride Citrate prescription drug users getting their prescription filled locally?

Notes:

81. Are any nutrients depleted by this Mosapride Citrate medication?

Notes:

82. Will I be able to do _____ after treatment?

Notes:

83. Why is buying Mosapride Citrate prescription drugs without a prescription dangerous?

Notes:

84. Can I take Mosapride Citrate with prescription medication or with an underlying medical condition?

Notes:

85. Why are Mosapride Citrate medications so popular?

Notes:

86. Are my Mosapride Citrate medications safe to use while breastfeeding?

Notes:

87. They say _____ not to take this with Mosapride Citrate prescription medication, but do you think it will hurt me?

Notes:

88. How will the treatment effect the medications that I currently take for _____?

Notes:

89. Could I have afforded it without Mosapride Citrate prescription drug insurance?

Notes:

90. Why go the Mosapride Citrate medication route?

Notes:

91. Do generic medications have the exact same ingredients?

Notes:

92. Will Mosapride Citrate medication control my symptoms adequately?

Notes:

93. Are herbal supplements safe when I am taking other Mosapride Citrate prescription medications?

Notes:

CHAPTER #6: HOW:

INTENT: How will Mosapride Citrate affect me (How will it affect me negatively. How do I know if its a problem for me.)

1. How long do I need to take the Mosapride Citrate medicine for?

Notes:

2. Are there drugs to lift my mood, and how can this be achieved without prescription medications?

Notes:

3. So how do I save money on my Mosapride Citrate prescription drugs?

Notes:

4. Is it probable to find out how to deal with my condition without taking Mosapride Citrate prescription drugs?

Notes:

5. How quickly do I have to start the treatment?

Notes:

6. Can I travel to _____ with prescription drugs used as medication for my condition?

Notes:

7. How do I know if I have permanent hair loss due to medication?

Notes:

8. Are there support groups for people with this problem and how would I contact them?

Notes:

9. How serious is this condition?

Notes:

10. How can I reduce or stop some of my medications?

Notes:

11. How long do I have to take Mosapride Citrate medication?

Notes:

12. How do I take this Mosapride Citrate medication?

Notes:

13. In case I need pain relief, how can I get access to medical cannabis?

Notes:

14. May an employer ask all employees what prescription medications they are taking?

Notes:

15. How soon should I come back?

Notes:

16. How do different Mosapride Citrate-class prescription medications work differently?

Notes:

17. How will Mosapride Citrate affect my sleeping pattern?

Notes:

18. How do generic medications compare in quality to brand name drugs?

Notes:

19. How do the police suspect impairment by Mosapride Citrate prescription medication?

Notes:

20. How to go about it if I want to use a lower dosage of Mosapride Citrate?

Notes:

21. Can I take this Mosapride Citrate medicine if I am pregnant?

Notes:

22. How can I find a few methods that can help my condition without the use of Mosapride Citrate prescription medication?

Notes:

23. How can I learn more about my symptoms or condition?

Notes:

24. How do I get better without Mosapride Citrate medication?

Notes:

25. How long will I need the treatment for?

Notes:

26. So I got a condition and a Mosapride Citrate medication – how am I, as a patient, supposed to manage treatment?

Notes:

27. Do you know how long it will take me to get my Mosapride Citrate medication?

Notes:

28. How will Mosapride Citrate affect the other medications that I'm taking?

Notes:

29. How many surgeries do you perform each year?

Notes:

30. How can Mosapride Citrate medication be detected?

Notes:

31. How to store Mosapride Citrate medication?

Notes:

32. How can I reduce my Mosapride Citrate prescription drug costs?

Notes:

33. How long does the prescription drug Mosapride Citrate stay in your system?

Notes:

34. How will I know if the Mosapride Citrate prescription and over-the-counter medications I take are interacting properly?

Notes:

35. How is the test done?

Notes:

36. How does Mosapride Citrate interact with other medications?

Notes:

37. How do we order or pick up Mosapride Citrate medications?

Notes:

38. So how do you know if you, or someone you love is having problems with Mosapride Citrate prescription drug abuse?

Notes:

39. How often do I need to have the test done?

Notes:

40. How long will it take to get the results?

Notes:

41. Is Mosapride Citrate as effective as other prescription medications?

Notes:

42. How do I dispose of Mosapride Citrate prescription medications?

Notes:

43. How long does a Mosapride Citrate medication remain active in your body?

Notes:

44. How does Mosapride Citrate prescription drug abuse start?

Notes:

45. How about a new Mosapride Citrate-like

prescription drug?

Notes:

46. Will grapefruit affect my Mosapride Citrate medications?

Notes:

47. How can my mental state successfully improve using medication or therapy?

Notes:

48. How can I make sure I am sufficiently stocked with the Mosapride Citrate prescription medications I need?

Notes:

49. Have you instructed patients to discontinue taking their Mosapride Citrate, or other prescription drugs?

Notes:

50. How long is it likely to last?

Notes:

51. Are there any other restrictions on Mosapride Citrate prescription drug coverage?

Notes:

52. How is the Mosapride Citrate medication delivered?

Notes:

53. Are Mosapride Citrate medications safe for young kids?

Notes:

54. How long should I take Mosapride Citrate medication?

Notes:

55. Are these Mosapride Citrate medications really helping?

Notes:

56. How effective is this treatment?

Notes:

57. How can I opt for the generic alternative Mosapride Citrate medication that gives me the exact same results?

Notes:

58. How soon do I need to have the test?

Notes:

59. How accurate are the results of the test?

Notes:

60. How do I manage my Mosapride Citrate medications?

Notes:

61. How should I take my Mosapride Citrate medication?

Notes:

62. How should I use this Mosapride Citrate medication?

Notes:

63. How do you handle children on Mosapride Citrate medication?

Notes:

64. How long will the effect of Mosapride Citrate medication last?

Notes:

65. How's my weight?

Notes:

66. State prescription drug price web sites, how useful

are they to me as a Mosapride Citrate consumer?

Notes:

67. How does a person with dementia, living alone, manage her Mosapride Citrate medication?

Notes:

68. How often is the Mosapride Citrate medication taken?

Notes:

69. How should I dispose of Mosapride Citrate prescription drugs?

Notes:

70. Should I take medication to lower my blood pressure?

Notes:

71. How will I know if my current Mosapride Citrate Prescription Drug coverage is as good as the new

Medicare Mosapride Citrate Prescription Drug coverage?

Notes:

72. Is it legal to buy Mosapride Citrate prescription medications online?

Notes:

73. How can I support my bone health naturally with and without medication?

Notes:

74. How are Mosapride Citrate prescription drugs abused?

Notes:

75. How will I get the test results?

Notes:

76. How do I read the label on my Mosapride Citrate prescription drug package?

Notes:

77. How do I manage multiple prescription medications together with Mosapride Citrate?

Notes:

78. How common is Mosapride Citrate prescription drug abuse?

Notes:

79. How should this Mosapride Citrate medication be taken?

Notes:

80. How is Mosapride Citrate medication supposed to help me?

Notes:

81. My Mosapride Citrate medications, just how safe are they?

Notes:

82. How will I hear about my test results?

Notes:

83. How often will I take the Mosapride Citrate medication?

Notes:

84. How long does the Mosapride Citrate medication last?

Notes:

85. Is it necessary to refill my Mosapride Citrate medication repeatedly annually?

Notes:

86. I am on prescription Mosapride Citrate medication, can I still detox?

Notes:

87. How should I take this Mosapride Citrate medication?

Notes:

88. How can I dispose of my Mosapride Citrate prescription drugs safely?

Notes:

89. How can Mosapride Citrate prescription drug abuse be recognized and stopped?

Notes:

90. How should this Mosapride Citrate medication be stored?

Notes:

91. How will I feel when I'm on Mosapride Citrate medications?

Notes:

92. How many patients with my condition have you treated?

Notes:

93. How wide-ranging is the Mosapride Citrate prescription drug coverage?

Notes:

CHAPTER #7: HOW MUCH:

INTENT: How much will taking Mosapride Citrate cost me (In money and Mosapride Citrate's effect on quality of life.)

1. Where can one undertake Mosapride Citrate prescription drug addiction treatment?

Notes:

2. Should I take Mosapride Citrate with food or drink?

Notes:

3. How much do I need to really understand about the interactions of my Mosapride Citrate prescription drugs?

Notes:

4. How much will the plan cover for Mosapride Citrate prescription drugs?

Notes:

5. What are the active ingredients in Mosapride Citrate prescription medication?

Notes:

6. Is there an alternative medication?

Notes:

7. How much will the treatment cost?

Notes:

8. How much am I likely to spend on Mosapride Citrate prescription drugs?

Notes:

9. Could theMosapride Citrate prescription drug I am taking now be the cause of a few extra pounds?

Notes:

10. Is this necessary right now?

Notes:

11. Just how much do you know about the numerous types of Mosapride Citrate medications for the different types of my condition?

Notes:

12. Are all Mosapride Citrate drugs covered by my prescription drug benefit?

Notes:

13. How much should I be charged for my Mosapride Citrate prescription medications?

Notes:

14. Which medication for my condition is right for

me?

Notes:

15. Are there generic equivalents available for my Mosapride Citrate prescription drugs?

Notes:

16. How much is Medicare Mosapride Citrate prescription drug coverage worth?

Notes:

17. Can Mosapride Citrate medications or my health problems keep me awake?

Notes:

18. Is it covered by Medicare - my concession or Veterans Affairs card or my private health insurance?

Notes:

19. Do I really need this treatment?

Notes:

20. What if I take pain medication for _____?

Notes:

21. Is Mosapride Citrate compatible with my current prescribed medication?

Notes:

22. Which part of Medicare will cover my Mosapride Citrate prescription drugs?

Notes:

23. Is there financial help for Mosapride Citrate prescription drugs?

Notes:

24. Should I join a Medicare Prescription Drug Plan even if I don't take many prescription drugs?

Notes:

25. Can enzymes be taken when a person is on Mosapride Citrate prescription medications?

Notes:

26. How much Mosapride Citrate prescription medication can I order from my pharmacy at one time?

Notes:

27. How does a Mosapride Citrate medication reminder service work?

Notes:

28. What do you turn to for adjunctive medications, usually?

Notes:

29. Is Mosapride Citrate safe if taking medications for high blood pressure?

Notes:

30. How much will my Mosapride Citrate prescription drugs cost me?

Notes:

31. How much Mosapride Citrate medication can be brought through customs in case I travel?

Notes:

32. Would using Mosapride Citrate mean that I would need my other medications less?

Notes:

33. What should I do if my symptoms are not relieved while taking Mosapride Citrate medication?

Notes:

34. I am feeling anxious and/or blue lately. Is this normal, can you help me?

Notes:

35. How much does it normally cost to get the surgery done, including all Mosapride Citrate medications and tests (ultrasounds,x-rays,medicines, hospital stay)?

Notes:

36. Is the Mosapride Citrate medication safe?

Notes:

37. Can you explain my options for Medicare, Medicare/Medicaid, Disability, Supplemental Insurance, Part D Prescription Drug Plans, or Medicare Billings?

Notes:

38. Is there a Medicare Advantage plan provider who will cover my Mosapride Citrate prescription drug costs during the donut hole?

Notes:

39. What are the effects of Mosapride Citrate medications on cognition?

Notes:

40. Will the cost be covered by Medicare - my concession or Veterans Affairs card or by private health insurance?

Notes:

41. How much can I use this Mosapride Citrate prescription drug plan?

Notes:

42. Can I still take my current medications?

Notes:

43. Are all drug-drug interactions limited to Mosapride Citrate prescription medications?

Notes:

44. Am I am worrying too much?

Notes:

45. Should I review my Medicare prescription drug plan choice every year?

Notes:

46. How do prescription medications compare to herbal forms of treatment for my condition?

Notes:

47. How much will this cost me?

Notes:

48. Should I bring a copy of my prescription medications?

Notes:

49. Can I drink alcohol while I am taking Mosapride Citrate?

Notes:

50. Which Mosapride Citrate-like medication gives the most rapid relief?

Notes:

51. Regarding dosage, exactly how much of Mosapride Citrate can I take?

Notes:

52. I am paid to _____ for a living, will my performance improve or decrease while using Mosapride Citrate prescription drugs?

Notes:

53. How will I know when my Mosapride Citrate medications are working?

Notes:

54. Which prescription medications can cause impotence?

Notes:

55. How much will the test cost?

Notes:

56. So, is this a 'wow-factor' Mosapride Citrate medication?

Notes:

57. Are nutritional supplements safe to take if I am taking Mosapride Citrate prescription medications?

Notes:

58. How much do the Mosapride Citrate prescription drugs cost in this plan as compared to other plans?

Notes:

59. I Googled my symptoms and read this. Is it accurate?

Notes:

60. How much will it cost, will the cost be covered by the PBS - my concession or Veterans Affairs card

or by private health insurance?

Notes:

61. How do I know how much my Mosapride Citrate prescription medication will be?

Notes:

62. Can my child have his or her Mosapride Citrate medication administered during the school day?

Notes:

63. Are there any risks involved in having this test?

Notes:

64. Are there any counter-indications about taking this supplement while taking any prescription drugs?

Notes:

65. Can or should I take my Mosapride Citrate medications at breakfast with my grapefruit juice?

Notes:

66. Will these Mosapride Citrate medications cause weight gain?

Notes:

67. How long will I need to take this Mosapride Citrate medication?

Notes:

68. Are medication reminders only for prescription medications?

Notes:

69. Are there other ways to treat my condition?

Notes:

70. How much does Mosapride Citrate cost?

Notes:

71. Can anyone get these Mosapride Citrate prescription drugs?

Notes:

72. Which of my medications cause the most weight gain?

Notes:

73. Will my Mosapride Citrate prescription drug have a drivers warning on it?

Notes:

74. Will any of the supplements that have been prescribed for me interfere with any Mosapride Citrate prescription medications I may already be on?

Notes:

75. Who typically, signed up for the Medicare Prescription Drug plan, are already hitting the gap in coverage known as the doughnut hole - and what is my risk of hitting the doughnut hole?

Notes:

76. Will Mosapride Citrate interact with any other medicines I take - including any vitamins - herbal medicine or other complementary medicine?

Notes:

77. If I get sick - will you see me in the hospital?

Notes:

78. Are there any risks or side effects?

Notes:

79. I take daily prescription medications, may I take my pills before I have my blood drawn?

Notes:

80. Can my Mosapride Citrate medication be delivered if I don't attend appointments?

Notes:

81. Are there any supplements or Mosapride Citrate medications?

Notes:

82. Am I up to date on my routine health maintenance?

Notes:

83. Can I take _____ with Mosapride Citrate prescription drugs?

Notes:

84. Can certain over the counter medications or Mosapride Citrate prescription medications cause a false positive for illegal drugs in a blood test?

Notes:

85. Will it help when I tell you about all my current medications and vitamin and herbal supplements?

Notes:

86. What is this Mosapride Citrate medication for, why am I taking it?

Notes:

87. Can natural be just as potent, if not more potent than over-the-counter drugs, creams and ointments?

Notes:

88. How do I get the Medicare Mosapride Citrate prescription drug benefit?

Notes:

89. Will Medicare be enough to cover the cost of my medical care, especially Mosapride Citrate prescription drugs?

Notes:

90. Are my prescription drugs also available in a generic version?

Notes:

91. Can I use this app I found?

Notes:

92. How much experience with this test or procedure do you have?

Notes:

93. Can I take the generic version of your prescription drugs?

Notes:

Index

happen   19, 47, 49, 55
happens   38-39, 43, 50, 57, 63
harmed   22
harmful   28, 34
harmless   70
having 3, 24, 51, 106, 121, 145
healing   48
health 1, 3-5, 21, 31, 55, 63-65, 67, 92, 96, 98, 100, 128, 136, 141, 145, 149
healthy   44
helping   124
herbal 25, 80, 82, 113, 142, 148-149
herein 1
higher 8
highlight   4
history 61, 97
hitting 147
hospital   140, 148
identified   1
illegal 11, 149
impairment   117
important   3-5, 29, 37, 102
impotence   12, 143
improve   3, 14, 62, 89, 123, 143
include   94
included   31, 107
including   61, 140, 148
increase   99
increased   15
increasing   69
indirectly   1
individual   21
influence   58
inform 70
informed   1
instead70, 106
instructed   123
insurance   8, 28, 87, 96, 107, 112, 136, 140-141, 145
insurers 100
intended   1
INTENT 7, 26, 57, 76, 95, 114, 133
intention   1
interact   24, 32, 37, 60, 84, 97, 121, 148